Mediterranean Diet:

How to Permanently Lose Weight and Lower the Risk of Heart Disease, Plus 38 Amazing Recipes

By Brianna Simmons

in the rendering of legal, financial, medical or professional advice.

By reading this document, the reader agrees that under no circumstances are we responsible for any losses, direct or indirect, which are incurred as a result of the use of information contained within this document, including, but not limited to; errors, omissions, or inaccuracies.

Table of Contents

Introduction

Back in the 1960s, people in the Mediterranean were observed to be living a lot healthier than Americans and other natives from other countries of the same age. They were also less susceptible to many killer diseases and illnesses. Since the 1960s and to the current times, many studies have been carried out. The research definitively shows, that the Mediterranean diet can: help with weight loss, aid in the prevention of heart attacks, strokes and type 2 diabetes. All of which can all lead to premature death and or decreased quality of life.

The diet is a heart-healthy eating plan which aims to fulfill your appetite, rather than make you feel deprived after or between meal times. Most healthy diets are based on whole grains, fruit, vegetables, and fish. After careful analysis, it has been shown, with minor variations in the quantities of the proportions of some foods - the risk of heart disease can be reduced, massively.

A lot of diets aim to reduce fats and oils in the diet, but the Mediterranean diet actually encourages both (in small amounts). So, to follow the characteristics of Mediterranean cooking, and also have the ability to have meals with friends is a bonus! Many of them may not even realize you are on a diet. Throughout the book, I will give you all that you need to know about feeling healthy and revived through correct eating, the Mediterranean way...

Chapter 1: Eating the Mediterranean Way

The Mediterranean is a large area consisting of many different countries, so not all the same foods are eaten by the same nationalities, which shows us that the benefits are not only coming from certain foods in this diet. Actually, the benefits are coming from eating a certain way and the foods together. This can vastly increase what types of foods you can eat, and not leave you with a limited grocery list, during the process.

I will explain in more detail what the Mediterranean diet consists of and the what you can eat (including the things that you must limit or avoid altogether). So please remember that all the information given is only a guideline, and the plans and recipes given can be adjusted for your personal preferences. As with all diets, if you have any doubts or are on any medication, always consult your doctor before commencement.

Regular Eating

Vegetables: Cucumber, Carrots, Cauliflower, Tomatoes, Broccoli, Kale, Onions and Spinach plus others.

Seeds and Nuts: Almonds, Walnuts, Sunflower, Pumpkin and Cashews etc.

Tubers: Potatoes, Turnips and Sweet Potatoes etc.

Poultry: Chicken, Turkey or Duck.

Whole Grains: Whole Grain Bread, Pasta, Barley, Corn and Brown Rice plus others.

Note: in the Mediterranean, bread is normally only used for dipping and not used in sandwiches.

Herbs and Spices: Garlic, Rosemary, Sage, Pepper etc.

Fish and Seafood: Mackerel, Trout, Salmon, Shrimp, Prawns, Mussels etc.

Fruits: Apples, Oranges, Pears, Figs, Dates, Avocados and any Berries plus many more.

Legumes: Beans, Peas, Lentils and Chickpeas etc.

Good Fats and Oils: Extra Virgin Olive Oil and Olives, Avocado Oil.

Moderate Eating

Yogurt, cheese, poultry and eggs.

Less frequent eating and red meats.

Things to Avoid

Processed foods – Low fat, diet or ready meals.

Processed meats – Hot dogs or sausages etc.

Trans fats – These are found in processed foods and margarine.

Refined grains – Anything made with refined wheat, white bread, pasta etc.

Refined oils – Canola oil, soybean oil etc.

Sugary things – Sugar for tea, coffee, sodas, candy, ice cream.

Drinks

Compared to most diets, coffee and tea are accepted and the recommended amount of red wine per day is one glass. Water should be consumed throughout the day to keep you hydrated, plus it helps to flush out your system. Fruit Juices and sweetened drinks should be avoided as they contain extra sugar.

Snacks

With the Mediterranean way of eating you normally only eat three times per day, although if you get hungry between meals here are a few things that you can have as a snack: half a cup of nuts, half a cup of berries, raw carrots, and fruit.

Dining Out on the Mediterranean Diet

If dining out at restaurants, you will probably realize this is one of the easiest diets cater for, so here are a few tips on how to make your meal suitable.

Order whole grain bread and instead of butter ask if they have olive oil for spreading. Ask if they can fry your food in olive oil, or if there is the possibility of having the food steamed. Choose fish or seafood for your main course.

The general principles are not to give a quick fix or to starve your body of certain foods that are required for normal day to day activity. The purpose is to give healthy eating on a daily basis - this of which has no adverse effects if followed over the long term like some diets.

As a general rule, you should aim to maximize your intake of any of the foods that are in the eat frequently section e.g. fruits, vegetables, legumes and wholegrain cereals. Limit the amount of salt used for flavoring when cooking, because the increased amount has been directly linked to high blood pressure. The alternatives to flavoring by using salt are herbs and spices, and also garlic.

The countries in the Mediterranean include Greece, Spain and southern Italy being the main ones. After you have seen and tried some of the recipes in this book, it is simple to find more healthy variations from these countries. So, you will soon realize with a slight adaption they can fit into your diet with ease as most recipes are already diet friendly. You will also notice the recipes contain high amounts of legume consumption, this is recommended on a regular level along with unrefined cereals, fruits and vegetables, especially leafy green vegetables, too. And all of them have increased amounts of olive oil, either for cooking or to add flavor to your dishes.

You will also notice, most recipes call for fish or seafood, and this is recommended above poultry and red meats. Many studies have shown the main contributing factor to the benefits of the diet is actually the olive oil, of which you should aim to use Extra Virgin Olive Oil, where possible. And although slightly more expensive, it is a much higher quality - as it is the purest oil that comes from the first pressing of the olives. It is said that olive oil may lower the risks of all mortality cancers, cardiovascular disease and other chronic diseases, as well.

Although there are many countries around the Mediterranean, this diet takes a broad overview of foods and recipes available from all these countries plus others. I have tried to not limit the recipes to one particular country. You will also notice you can have 2 small glasses of red wine or 1 large glass per day, and studies show that this can also help decrease the risk of heart disease, stroke, diabetes and early death.

Please note, drinking more than this amount can actually increase the risks of the illnesses that a small amount helps to cure. Although this diet has been around for many years, there is the Mediterranean Diet Foundation which is based in Barcelona, where they still continue to study the benefits of the Mediterranean diet. It is also important to note that their aim is to promote investigation of health, historical, cultural and gastronomic aspects of the Mediterranean Diet. As with their own studies, they also analyze the scientific results of tests that others have conducted, in accordance to regulatory guidelines. It shows how important the people of the Mediterranean take this diet, as this foundation was first established in 1996.

If you are interested, you can search for more exclusive information regarding this amazing diet online. Sometimes you need to see the results or stories of others to believe that they are true. In saying that, there are also well backed research results which can be looked at in conjunction with this information. I want you to have the entire picture, so you can see for yourself.

Chapter 2: A Successful Plan for You

With most diets, you are encouraged to do regular exercise which helps to burn calories. Not only is this tiring and time consuming but it is also slightly misleading, because the benefits you are getting are from the diet and not just from extra exercise you are doing. As the Mediterranean diet is a well-balanced diet without many food items having to be omitted, you do not have to do much additional exercise to what you would normally do, although it is recommended to have an exercise regime in place or to keep physically active, for health promotion.

Although after a while you will be doing this anyway, as you will feel more energetic naturally. As the majority of the food items on the Mediterranean diet are fruits and vegetables (with limited amounts of red meats and dairy and poultry), most of these are absorbed and digested by the body a lot quicker, so not only are the nutrients absorbed faster, but there will be nothing making you feel overly bloated after meal times.

The best way to plan your diet is on a weekly basis, this way you can easily monitor your intake of dairy and red meats, these you can save for dining out with friends to make you evening more enjoyable. When planning your meals, you should choose a varied menu and try to include fish and seafood two to three times per week if not more. Iron would be substituted via vitamins, if you are anemic.

To keep physically active, it is recommended you either start a new sport or go dancing, there is no need for strenuous trips to the gym. To make this easier it is best to enlist the help of a partner or a friend, as this will take away the thought of starting something new with a lot of strangers.

A few sample exercises you can do at home are:

Bodyweight Squats

Stand as straight as you can with feet apart slightly wider than shoulder width. Hold arms straight in front of you at shoulder level.

Brace your abs and lower your body as far as you can by bending your knees.

Repeat a few times until you can do it more easily and then do about 20 repetitions.

Hip Raise

Lay flat on the floor with your knees bent and your feet are flat, and place your arms at a 45-degree angle with palms facing up.

Hold your stomach in and hold it in, this gives you a tight core, and breathe normally and then raise your hips so your body forms a straight line when raised. Pause for 5 seconds then lower back to the starting position. Once you have got used to this, do 10 repetitions at a time.

These are just a couple of easy exercises you can do a couple of times per day as they don't take too much time to do, maybe 15 minutes in a morning and 15 minutes in an evening. This would be the full allocation of exercise that is recommended on a daily basis, and that is without too much exertion or without any other activities you do.

Time Management

As we have mentioned, the Mediterranean diet will lead to a change in eating habits and lifestyle and is generally based on 3 good meals a day. For this reason, you should aim to give yourself time to actually fit these meal times into your day. If you are extra busy and only have time for a snack, you will feel deprived after eating. So you will become hungry before your next meal and will have the urge to snack, not only this, you will have missed out on the nutrients that one of the lunch dishes would have given you.

When doing your weekly plan, if you can allocate the times for your morning exercise, breakfast, lunch, dinner and evening activities and stick to this, the whole routine will become a habit. Not only will you feel better and less hungry, but you will start to do these things without having to think about it - so you will have less urge to snack in between meals. The other benefit of sticking to your routine is, if you happen to slip on your meals or routine, it will not have as much effect, if it occurs sometimes. Always try to keep your routine, though.

Staying Focused

In the start as with most diets, you can be tempted to slip - which would lead to quitting all your hard work. When and if you find yourself hungry between meals it is recommended to have a piece of fruit or a small handful of nuts - as these are on your, "eat regularly" list of foods. Other tips are to drink lots of water throughout the day, as this will keep you hydrated and also stave off hunger.

If you are on the Mediterranean diet with the aim to lose weight, try not to weigh yourself daily and only do it once per week if you must. Your body can fluctuate throughout the day, especially if you have been drinking lots of water, and this would still be in your system and show up when you are on the scales. Aim to get a good night's sleep, and remember that sitting on the couch and watching too much TV gives unnecessary distractions. This may lead into the temptation to snack, even if you are not really hungry. Chewing sugarless chewing gum is also another tip to stop you feeling hungry, as this will keep your mind and mouth occupied. One final tip is to keep a diary of everything that you eat and drink, this will make you aware of how much you are physically consuming. Also, studies have shown people who keep a diary tend to lose more weight than people who don't.

As a final comment, you should try to enjoy your diet and don't think of it as a chore that has to be done, if it is enjoyable it will become easier. So make it fun, and have fun while you do it. It can be a total lifestyle change, which is recommended for longevity in health, and for your heart, as well.

Chapter 3: Adapting the Perfect Diet Plan

As the Mediterranean diet is primarily a vegetable and fruit diet it is quite easy to adapt to, for meals not containing meat. Meals containing meat can be altered to use legumes, and more nuts and seeds and soy based products. The diet pyramid also puts emphasis on whole grains as part of the daily diet with fats playing a small part. If you adapt the diet for no meat, it is advisable to increase your intake of unsalted nuts to one handful per day - to counteract the loss of protein you would be getting from fish and poultry etc. You could also use dried beans, tempeh or tofu based products and also non-fat dairy products. It is also recommended to eat your maximum allocation of eggs and cheese on a daily or weekly basis.

Some considerations must be noted, if your diet consists of no meat or fish, it is also advisable to take fish oil supplements to boost your intake of omega-3 fatty acids which are found in seafood, because this also helps maintain the cardiovascular benefits you will gain from being on the Mediterranean diet. As you will lose some vitamin D, it is advisable to make sure all the dairy products you consume are fortified with Vitamin D, and also combine your bean dishes with generous servings of leafy green vegetables and tomatoes. The extra vitamin C you will gain from the vegetables helps to absorb the iron that is provided by the beans. Spending more time in sunlight will also increase your intake of vitamin D. As a general rule, vegetarians that are on the Mediterranean diet should aim to have at least six portions of fruit and vegetables per day, with whole grain cereals, bread and pasta eaten at every meal.

As it is advised throughout the diet, you should omit the use of butter and instead replace it with olive oil when cooking - or use it to flavor bread and also as a combination which can be used as a dip.

If you are vegetarian it is advisable to pay a visit to your doctor before commencing, so they can advise what you can do to boost your intake of vitamin B-12.

If you are vegan and also wish to try the Mediterranean diet, this is also possible and easy to adapt the recipes to include no animal products. Some recommendations are as follows:

Have larger servings of whole grains and vegetables, beans are of a significant importance as they lower blood cholesterol levels and are linked to improved blood glucose. Add a little extra virgin olive oil onto your vegetables which can help with the absorption of some compounds.

Flavor your dishes by using nuts and seeds, as this also adds texture so your mouthfuls are more interesting. Herbs and spices can improve flavor and also provide protective phytonutrients.

For your food supplements consider DHA and EPA, these are long chain Omega-3 fatty acids which are found in fatty fish.

These can also be purchased in non-gel capsules with the nutrients coming from algae-based products - which contain no traces of animal products. As with the vegetarians, it is advisable to keep active, enjoy the sunlight and make the most of your healthy lifestyle.

If you like meat in your diet it is advisable to follow what is laid out in the food pyramid and limit your red meat intake. Then when you do this, your portion of meat should only be the size of a pack of playing cards. It is also recommended not to eat fatty meats like sausages and bacon, as this type of fat are non-healthy fats and have no benefit to your system (and just lay in your stomach).

It is highly recommended you swap some of your red meat meals for poultry dishes, although these are recommended to be limited, so the best solution is to increase the amount of seafood and fish you consume, and save your red meat or poultry dish for special occasions. Or incorporate them only twice or three times per week, essentially.

Chapter 4: Beautiful Breakfast Recipes

Sparta Oatmeal

Serves 1

Ingredients

¼ cup cut oats

1 sprig parsley (chopped)

4 dates (chopped)

3 tbsp. olive oil

Salt and pepper (to taste)

¼ cup shallots (chopped)

2 slices tofu, 2 cups dates

Bacon 2 slices

Instructions

Cook the oats by instructions on the packet, sauté the shallots, bacon, and shallots, until soft, add rosemary and stir until all mixture is combined add salt and pepper to taste.

Transfer to dish.

Serve warm.

Chickpea Hash Browns

Serves 2

Ingredients

2 cups frozen hash browns

¼ cup chopped onion

¼ tsp salt

2 large eggs organic or free range

½ tbsp. ginger minced or grated

1/8 cup extra virgin olive oil

7 ½ oz. (½ can) chickpeas

½ cup zucchini chopped

1 tsp chili (can also use curry powder ½ tbsp.)

1 cup finely chopped leafy greens (kale, baby spinach or cabbage can be used)

Instructions

In a large bowl combine the hash browns, leafy greens, ginger, chili powder, and salt.

Heat oil in a skillet over medium heat.

Add mixture and press until level and flat.

Cook until golden brown on the bottom.

Reduce heat to low temperature.

Break the potato mixture then add the zucchini and chickpeas until combined.

Press flat again and make 4 indentations in the mixture.

Crack eggs and pour 1 into each dent, cover and cook until eggs are set. This should be 4 – 5 minutes for runny yolks.

Greek Honey Yogurt with Dates

Serves 1

Ingredients

1 small carton Greek yogurt

¼ cup pitted dates chopped

1 tbsp. honey

Instructions

Place yogurt in small dish.

Pour on chopped dates and combine.

Drizzle with honey.

Whole Grain Healthy Pancakes

Makes 2 large pancakes – double quantities to make more

Ingredients

½ cup oats

½ tsp baking soda

1/8 tsp salt

1 tbsp. canola oil

1 tbsp. honey (agave can be used)

1 cup Greek-style yogurt (either plain or vanilla)

1 large egg

¼ cup all-purpose flour

1 tbsp. flax seeds

Optional for Toppings

Fruit or syrup or any other from your allowed foods.

Instructions

In a blender pulse the oats, flour, flax seeds, baking soda and salt for about 30 seconds.

Add the yogurt and egg, oil and honey then blend until you have a smooth batter.

Let batter stand for about 20 minutes or until thickened.

Heat a non-stick skillet over medium heat and coat surface thinly with oil.

Pour half the mixture into the skillet and cook until golden brown on the bottom and bubbles start to form on the top surface approx. 2 minutes. Flip your pancake and cook for another 2 minutes.

Cook remaining half of the batter then transfer to plates and serve warm with your toppings, re-oil pan if required.

If pancakes are too large, just reduce quantity into the skillet, approx. ¼ cup.

Greek Yoghurt and Berry Surprise

Serves 1

Ingredients

6 oz. Greek yogurt

¼ cup berries

3 tbsp. low fat granola

honey

Instructions

In a tall glass place 1/3 of the yogurt followed by 1 tbsp. granola and cover with berries.

Cover berries with yogurt and granola.

Repeat until you have used all the ingredients then drizzle with honey.

Oatmeal with Banana and Nut Topping

Ingredients

2 peeled bananas

4 tbsp. chopped walnuts or almonds any other nuts can be used

½ cup cooking oats

1 cup skimmed milk

2 tsp flax seeds

6 tbsp. honey

Instructions

Place in a microwave safe bowl the bananas and mash with a fork.

Add milk, cooking oats, flax seeds, nuts and honey, stir mixture until well combined.

Cook in microwave on high for 2 minutes.

Divide into bowls and serve hot.

Toastie with Avocado

Serves 1

Ingredients

2 large slices whole grain bread

1 small avocado

Lemon juice (to taste)

40 grams of feta cheese (crumbled)

2 thin slices ham

1 egg (organic or free range)

Fresh herbs (any of your choice)

Instructions

In a bowl place the avocado and smash with a fork, add lemon juice to taste.

Toast bread until golden then spoon mixture onto the toast, top with the cheese and ham and serve hot.

If using egg, place on top of ham and garnish with fresh herbs.

Cinnamon and Fruity Couscous

Makes 2

Ingredients

½ cup uncooked couscous (whole-wheat)

1 ½ cups low-fat milk

2 tsp olive oil

2-inch cinnamon stick (or cinnamon powder to taste)

3 tsp dark brown sugar

1/8 tsp salt

1/8 cup currants or raisins

¼ cup dried fruit chopped

Instructions

In a large saucepan heat milk and cinnamon on medium- high heat until small bubbles start to form around the edge.

Remove from heat and stir in couscous, currants, dried fruit of choice and 2 tsp of the sugar and the salt.

Cover and stand for 15 minutes.

If using cinnamon stick remove and divide into bowls, top with remaining butter and sugar, serve immediately.

Flavorsome Feta Frittata

Ingredients

½ cup crumbled feta cheese

3 tbsp. grated parmesan cheese

½ cup chopped red peppers

1 cup chopped onion

2 cloves grated or minced garlic

3 tbsp. olive oil

8 large organic or free-range eggs (beaten)

¼ cup half and half light cream and full fat milk

½ cup pitted olives

¼ cup fresh basil (chopped)

½ tsp ground black pepper

½ cup crushed onion and garlic flavored croutons

Instructions

Preheat broiler to temperature, medium high.

In broiler proof skillet heat oil and sauté onion and garlic until tender.

In large bowl beat eggs and the half and half.

Stir in peppers, olives, basil black pepper and feta cheese.

Pour mixture over the onion and garlic cook over medium heat until mixture starts to set.

Lift edge of frittata from side of skillet so wet mixture can run underneath, continue cooking until all mixture is nearly set, top most surface will still be moist, lower heat to avoid burning.

In a small bowl, crush the croutons and parmesan cheese with the remaining oil, sprinkle over the top of the frittata and broil on the top half of broiler until the top surface has set and the crouton crumbs are golden brown.

Divide between plates and serve hot.

Chapter 5: Sumptuous Snacks

Salad Skewers

Ingredients

1/3 cup olives

1/3 cup grape tomatoes small cherry tomatoes can be used

¼ seedless cucumber

Cocktail sticks

Instructions

On each cocktail stick, place 1 olive, 1 tomato and ½ slice of cucumber.

Serve with your favorite dip.

Dip in a Glass

Ingredients

3 oz. Greek yogurt plain

1 tbsp. fresh parsley chopped finely

½ cup humus

1 tsp lemon juice

2 medium tomatoes (de-seeded and chopped)

1/3 cup cucumber (de-seeded and chopped)

1/3 cup green olives (chopped)

¼ cup feta cheese (crumbled)

1 pinch salt

3 tbsp. onion (chopped)

Sliced veggies or whole meal pita bread (to be used for dipping)

Instructions

Into each serving glass layer 2 tbsp. humus, 1 tbsp. tomato, 1 tbsp. cucumber, 1 tbsp. olives and half tbsp. onion and top with 1 large tbsp. of yogurt mixture.

In a small bowl mix feta cheese, parsley, lemon juice, salt and yogurt.

Serve with vegetable strips and pita slices.

Crunchy Crackers with Feta

Ingredients

Black pepper to taste

Pinch of red pepper flakes

Garlic 2 cloves thinly sliced

Pitted olives 1 cup sliced

Feta cheese ½ cup diced

Olive oil 2 tbsp.

Lemon zest and juice of 1 lemon

Rosemary 1 tsp fresh and chopped

Instructions

In a bowl mix all the ingredients, cover and place in the refrigerator for up to one day.

When ready to serve, place a small spoonful on a whole wheat cracker.

Berry and Ricotta Tasty

Ingredients

Any berries ¾ cup

Ricotta cheese 2 tbsp.

Mixed nuts 1 tbsp. (toasted and crushed)

Instructions

Place nuts in food processor and pulse until fine crumbs appear.

Place berries in a microwave bowl.

Heat berries until warm 1 to 2 minutes.

Place ricotta cheese onto the warm berries and top with the crushed nuts.

Spiced Veggie Hummus Dips

Ingredients

1 tbsp. olive oil

1 small serving humus

1 medium carrot

½ medium cucumber

½ medium red bell pepper

1 pinch paprika

1 pinch cayenne pepper

Instructions

Place hummus in small serving bowl and stir in 1 pinch of paprika and 1 pinch of cayenne pepper. Add 1 tbsp. olive oil.

Peel carrot and slice thinly.

Cut the cucumber into thin strips.

De-seed 1 red pepper and slice 1 half into thin strips.

Dip vegetables in humus and enjoy.

Tasty Salad

Serves 4

Ingredients

1 head of lettuce (any variety of choice)

2 medium tomatoes (cut into wedges)

¼ cup pitted olives sliced (any variety of olives can be used)

¼ cup crumbled feta cheese

1 medium green pepper (de-seeded and thinly sliced)

1 medium red pepper (de-seeded and thinly sliced)

Salad Dressing

1 tbsp. olive oil

3 tbsp. lemon juice

½ tsp finely chopped oregano

½ tsp finely chopped cilantro

¼ tsp black pepper

Instructions

Prepare dressing – in a small jar combine lemon juice, olive oil, oregano, cilantro, and pepper and shake well.

Wash and dry lettuce leaves and place in salad bowl.

Add bell peppers, tomatoes, olives and feta cheese then pour over the dressing.

Gently toss to coat everything.

Tuna Pockets

Ingredients

1 whole wheat pitta bread

1 tbsp. olive oil

2 lettuce leaves any variety

¼ cucumber sliced

1 medium tomato sliced

1 small onion sliced

½ can tuna chunks

Salt to taste

Pepper to taste

Instructions

In a small bowl break the tuna chunks, add olive oil.

Toast pitta bread and cut into 2.

Open pitta bread and insert lettuce, tomato, cucumber and onion along with half the tuna.

Sprinkle with salt and pepper if required.

Chickpeas and Couscous

Ingredients

1/4 juiced lemon

2 tbsp. olive oil

1 tomato cut into wedges

1 small onion diced

¼ cucumber diced

7 oz. chickpeas

2 tbsp. olives

2 tbsp. fresh basil finely chopped

¼ cup uncooked couscous

Black pepper to taste

Instructions

Cook couscous as per instructions.

Add to mixing bowl then add tomato wedges, onion, cucumber, olives and chickpeas.

Pour over the olive oil and lemon juice and mix until combined.

Place into serving bowl and top with fresh basil.

Chapter 6: Magnificent Mains

Cheesy Baked Spinach

Makes 6

Ingredients

750 grams cooked and finely chopped spinach

200 grams of ricotta cheese

1 cup whole meal breadcrumbs

2 large organic eggs

1/3 cup sliced mushrooms

½ cup green bell peppers

1/2 cup sour cream

½ cup spaghetti sauce

250 grams of sliced mozzarella cheese

1 tsp basil

1/4 cup parmesan

Instructions

Cook and finely chop spinach.

In a large bowl, combine spinach, ricotta cheese, bread crumbs, eggs, mushrooms, and green peppers.

Preheat the oven to 350 degrees F.

Lightly brush a medium sized baking dish with olive oil and spread mixture evenly then spread sour cream on top.

Pour half of the spaghetti sauce across the top and spread with a spatula.

Cover with a layer of mozzarella cheese slices.

Spread remaining spaghetti sauce over cheese slices.

Sprinkle with basil and parmesan cheese.

Bake for 30 minutes.

Cauliflower Italian Style

Serves 4

Ingredients

1 head fresh cauliflower

1 green pepper (de-seeded and sliced)

2 tbsp. olive oil

125 grams of fresh mushrooms

2 tbsp. plain flour

1 cup milk

350 grams of pimento cheese

2 cloves minced garlic

Instructions

Preheat oven to 350 degrees F.

Place cauliflower florets in pan of boiling water and cook for 5 minutes, then drain.

In a skillet add small amount of olive oil and sauté the mushrooms, garlic, and peppers.

Remove skillet and add the flour a little at a time stirring rapidly, slowly add milk while stirring.

Return to the heat and while stirring, cook until mixture thickens.

Place cauliflower in ovenproof baking dish and lay slices of cheese on top then pour the creamed mixture on top of the cheese.

Bake for 20 minutes.

Oven Roasted Chicken Le Mediterranean

Ingredients

300 grams of chicken breast (skinless)

6 large tomatoes (halved)

1 medium onion

1 red bell pepper cut into chunks

¼ cup black olives

4 tbsp. olive oil

1 large courgette (sliced)

250 grams of potatoes (halved)

Salt and pepper (to taste)

1 large tbsp. pesto

Instructions

Preheat oven to 350 degrees F.

Lay all the vegetables in a flat baking dish the sprinkle over the olives.

Make cuts cross ways in the chicken breasts and lay on top of the vegetables.

Mix olive oil and pesto and spoon onto the chicken breasts.

Cover with foil and bake for 30 minutes.

Remove foil and cook for another 10 minutes until chicken is tender.

Serve warm.

South Med Shrimp

Ingredients

500 grams of shrimp fresh or frozen

1 tbsp. chopped finely parsley

1 small chopped onion

1 tbsp. chopped finely oregano

1 bay leaf

2 cloves minced garlic

3 tbsp. olive oil

¼ cup dry white wine

½ tsp salt

3 oz. crumbled Feta cheese

1 ½ tsp cornstarch

ground pepper to taste

1 large can crushed tomatoes

Instructions

Drain tomatoes and keep juice.

Heat skillet over medium heat, add olive oil and sauté the onion, garlic, and spices.

Add crushed tomatoes to skillet with the white wine, salt and pepper cook over high heat for 5 minutes.

Add cornstarch to the tomato juice then add to the skillet and stir, reduce heat and cook until sauce thickens.

Add shrimp and cook until they have turned pink and curled, remove from heat and mix in cheese.

Serve immediately.

Brown Rice with Feta Cheese

Ingredients

1 tsp olive oil

2 medium onions chopped

2 cups brown rice

6 cups vegetable stock

Salt to taste

1 lemon (juice and zest)

4 tbsp. feta cheese

3 spring onions (sliced)

1 tbsp. cilantro (chopped finely)

6 cloves garlic (minced)

Instructions

In a deep pan heat the oil over medium heat and sauté the garlic and onion for 3 minutes.

Add the rice and continue to cook while stirring until rice is coated in oil, about 2 minutes.

Add the vegetable stock while stirring and scraping the sides of the pan until rice starts to cook, season with salt to taste.

Cover and simmer on low heat for 25 minutes then remove from heat and allow to steam for 5 minutes.

Test rice for doneness, if liquid remains or rice is hard return to the heat for a few minutes.

Once cooked, add the feta cheese, spring onions, and cilantro, gently stir until combined.

Serve immediately.

Minestrone Stew

Serves 8

Ingredients

1 can drained kidney beans

2 cloves garlic chopped

Salt to taste

¼ tsp pepper

2 tbsp. olive oil

¼ cup parsley (chopped)

½ cup tomato juice (unsweetened)

1/3 cup whole wheat pasta

2 ½ cups water

1 small zucchini (chopped or sliced)

1 16 oz. can tomatoes

2 large celery stalks finely chopped (include leaves)

2 small diced carrots

1 small minced onion

2 medium diced potatoes

1 cup shredded cabbage

1 cup sliced green beans

Instructions

In a large pan add kidney beans and lightly squash with a fork.

Add garlic, pepper, oil, parsley and salt to taste stir well.

Add water and vegetables, bring to a boil and cook over medium heat while stirring.

Lower the heat, cover, and simmer for 1 hour.

Add pasta, tomato juice, and simmer for 15 minutes.

Salt to taste.

Mediterranean Meatballs

Serves 2

Ingredients

500 grams minced beef

1 tbsp. mint leaves

½ tsp dill dried flakes

½ tsp vinegar

3 cloves garlic (minced)

1 medium onion (finely chopped)

Salt to taste

Pepper to taste

2 slices whole meal bread

1 medium egg (beaten)

Sauce

8 oz. can unsweetened tomato sauce

1 small onion (chopped)

1/3 cup olive oil

1/8 tsp cloves

1/8 tsp nutmeg

1 bay leaf

Instructions

Mix all ingredients and form into small balls.

Flour lightly and lightly fry in a skillet until brown.

Add to sauce and simmer for 20 minutes, add water if needed.

Greek Chicken

Serves 6

Ingredients

1 kg chicken cut into serving sized pieces

3 tbsp. olive oil

5 cloves garlic

2 large onions (chopped)

3 cups Tomatoes (chopped)

¾ cup olives (any type of olives can be used)

Black pepper to taste

Salt to taste

2 tbsp. fresh oregano (or 1 tbsp. dried)

1 cup dry red wine

Instructions

In a skillet add olive oil, place chicken and cook on medium until brown.

Remove chicken and sauté the garlic and onions.

Add tomatoes and olives and cook until the tomatoes are soft, add pepper, oregano wine and chicken.

Cover and simmer for 30 minutes or until tender, taste for salt as the olives can affect the saltiness of the dish.

Serve warm.

Spicy Mediterranean Fillets

Serves 2

Ingredients

2 halibut fillets

1 large tomato (chopped)

¼ cup olives (any variety)

3 tbsp. olive oil

1 tbsp. lemon juice

Salt to taste

Pepper to taste

Parsley 2 tbsp. (chopped finely)

1 tsp cayenne pepper

Instructions

Heat oven to 350 degrees F.

Place fish fillet on a baking tray lined with aluminum foil and season with salt and pepper.

Combine tomato, olives, onion, olive oil, lemon juice in a bowl.

Sprinkle the fillet with cayenne pepper.

Spoon the mixture over the fish and then fold the foil and seal the edges making a large packet.

Bake on baking tray for 30 to 40 minutes.

When serving sprinkle with fresh parsley.

Mediterranean Spaghetti

4 tbsp. parmesan grated

Black pepper to taste

½ cup parsley chopped

½ cup breadcrumbs

2 cloves garlic crushed

3 tbsp. olive oil

500 grams of whole wheat spaghetti

½ can tuna chunks or flakes

Instructions

Cook spaghetti as per packet instructions until slightly al dente.

In a skillet heat olive oil and add garlic and anchovies, stir while cooking approx. 2 minutes.

Stir in breadcrumbs and remove from heat, add parsley and black pepper.

Toss anchovy sauce with hot pasta and sprinkle with cheese.

Serve warm.

Steamed Mussels

Serves 2

Ingredients

250 grams of mussels (cleaned)

1 tbsp. olive oil

1 clove garlic minced

½ can crushed tomatoes

¼ tsp dried oregano

¼ tsp dried basil

1 pinch red pepper flakes

¼ cup white wine

4 oz. whole wheat linguini pasta

½ lemon for garnish

Instructions

In a large skillet over medium heat sauté garlic and when soft add tomatoes, oregano, pepper flakes and basil lower heat then simmer for 5 minutes.

Cook pasta as per packet instructions or until slightly al dente.

Add mussels and wine to the skillet, cover and turn heat to high and cook for 4 – 5 minutes or until shells are open.

Pour over hot pasta and then sprinkle with parsley and lemon juice.

Chapter 7: Daring Desserts

Grilled Peaches with Mascarpone

Serves 2

Ingredients

1 large peach

120 grams of mascarpone cheese

1 tbsp. crushed nuts

Olive oil

Berries

1 large peach (cut in half with seed removed)

Instructions

Brush bottom of griddle pan with olive oil, brush flat surface of the peach halves.

Grill on one side only, when grill marks appear, transfer to serving plate, top with mascarpone cheese and berries and chopped nuts.

Sushi Dessert

Serves 2

Ingredients

1 large tbsp. pumpkin puree

1 medium orange (cut into 4 wedges)

2 sesame energy bars (orange and honey flavored)

Zest of 1 medium orange

2 tbsp. honey

2 tbsp. Greek yogurt

1 large tbsp. sesame paste (tahini)

Cinnamon to garnish

Instructions

In a food processor place pumpkin puree, yogurt, honey and orange zest, pulse until you have a smooth paste.

Place energy bars between two sheets of parchment paper on a flat surface, roll with rolling pin until it is about 2 mm thick.

Place half of the mixture onto each flat bar with a spoon and smooth out, roll the bars to form a round shape.

Cut into bite sized pieces and serve with orange wedges, honey and cinnamon.

Pudding-Rice with Fruit

Serves 4

Ingredients

½ cup basmati rice

3 tbsp. sugar

¼ cup chopped dates (raisins or currants can be used)

4 cups milk (for extra creaminess half and half can be used)

½ tsp cinnamon

1/8 tsp nutmeg

¼ cup nuts (almonds or walnuts chopped)

1 tbsp. orange zest

Instructions

Wash rice and drain.

In a large saucepan add milk and sugar and heat until milk starts to boil.

Add the rice, fruit and cinnamon and simmer over low heat for about 45 minutes, stir occasional.

Remove from heat, add chopped nuts and orange zest.

Pour into serving bowls and serve immediately.

Panna Delight

Serves 2

Ingredients

105 ml whipping cream

1 ½ tbsp. milk

1 tbsp. sugar

1 tbsp. honey

½ tsp gelatin

1 cup berries (any berries you prefer)

Instructions

Add a quarter of the cream to a small bowl and cover with the gelatin, allow to stand so the gelatin becomes soft.

In a saucepan add the remaining cream, milk, and sugar, slowly heat and bring to a boil while continuously stirring.

Remove from heat and whisk in the cream and gelatin mix until all the gelatin has dissolved.

Pour into 4 small containers and chill for at least 4 hours.

When ready to serve unmold onto serving plates.

Top with the berries and drizzle with the honey.

Italian Stuffed Apples

Serves 4

Ingredients

4 apples

1 tbsp. cinnamon powder

¼ cup (any dried fruit can be used depending on preference)

¼ cup brown sugar

Instructions

Preheat oven to 350 degrees F.

Wash and core the apples ¾ of the way so the bottom is still sealed.

Add quarter of the dried fruit to the hole in the apple and top with 1 tsp of the brown sugar then add 1 tsp cinnamon on top of the sugar.

Bake the apples for 1 hour.

Nut Peach Boats

Serves 4

Ingredients

4 peach halves (can use canned)

¼ cup (almonds or any other nuts)

½ ricotta cheese

2 tbsp. honey

¼ tsp cardamom

Instructions

Preheat oven to 400 degrees F.

Cut peaches in half and remove stone (if using fresh), rinse and place facing up onto a small baking sheet.

Mix ricotta cheese with honey and cardamom then spoon ¼ of the mixture into each peach.

Bake for 15 minutes.

Grind almonds in a food processor until fine crumbs have formed.

Gently toast in a pan over medium heat.

Remove peaches from oven and sprinkle with nut mixture.

Lemon Pudding

Serves 4

Ingredients

¾ cup sugar

2 lemons (zested)

2 lemons (juiced)

1 pinch salt

3 egg yolks (lightly beaten)

¼ cup cornstarch

2 tbsp. butter (unsalted at room temp)

2 ½ cups milk

½ cup heavy cream

¼ cup nuts (any variety)

Instructions

Add to a small bowl the sugar and cornstarch and whisk together, add milk and whisk until a smooth paste.

Add the egg yolks and whisk until completely combined.

Pour contents into a small saucepan stir and heat on medium until mixture thickens and sticks to the back of the spoon.

Remove from heat and combine the lemon juice and butter.

Once mixed divide between 4 small dishes.

Let cool and then cover with cling wrap and place in refrigerator to chill about 2 hours.

When ready to serve top with whipped cream and then sprinkle with nut crumbs.

Baklava with Cinnamon

Serves 6

Ingredients

9 sheets filo pastry

8 oz. mixed nuts (chopped finely)

1 tsp cinnamon

8 oz. butter (unsalted)

Syrup

125 ml honey

4 ½ oz. sugar

250 ml water

1 tsp vanilla

Instructions

Preheat oven to 350 degrees F.

Lightly grease a medium baking pan with butter.

Melt butter in a small pan over low heat.

Lay sheets to cover base of baking pan and brush with melted butter.

In a small bowl mix the mixed nuts and cinnamon.

Spread 3 tbsp. over the pastry sheets then cover with pastry sheets, once again brushing each with butter.

Repeat this until you have 2 pastry sheets remaining to cover the last layer of nut mixture.

Using a sharp knife cut a crisscross pattern into top layers of the pastry.

Place into heated oven and cook for about 40 minutes until pastry is puffed and golden on top.

Remove from oven and allow to cool slightly.

Syrup Instructions

In a small pan heat, the sugar, water, vanilla, and honey until the sugar has melted. This will take about 20 minutes stirring continuously to avoid burning.

Pour the syrup into the crisscross pattern you made and let stand to cool.

Cut into small pieces and serve.

Tiramisu

Serves 2

Ingredients

6 medium eggs

8 tbsp. caster sugar

10 tbsp. brandy

Cocoa powder

500 ml black coffee

8 ½ oz. mascarpone cheese

14 oz. sponge fingers

Instructions

Separate eggs and beat the yolks and sugar in a small bowl until thick.

In a separate bowl whisk egg whites until soft peaks form.

Add mascarpone cheese into yolk mixture and gently combine until you have a smooth mixture, now carefully fold in the beaten egg whites.

Mix brandy with the cold coffee into a shallow bowl, dip half of the sponge fingers into the coffee soaking both sides and then place into a dessert glasses or small bowls.

Divide half of the cheese mixture between the two glasses and smooth.

Dip the remaining sponge fingers dip into the coffee and divide between the two glasses.

Top with the remaining cheese mixture.

Chill for about 2 hours in the refrigerator.

When serving cover with cocoa powder.

Luscious Berries and Greek Yogurt

Serves 2

Ingredients

4 oz. Greek yogurt

1 cup Berries any variety

Nuts (any variety chopped finely)

2 tbsp. honey

Instructions

Divide yogurt between two small dishes, drizzle with 1 tbsp. honey and top with berries and chopped nuts.

Chapter 8: Long Term Weight Loss and Heart Smart Achievability

A lot of diets are designed to give a quick fix and rapid weight loss, and although you may be able to achieve your desired weight quickly, there is a good chance it will come back. Also, in following these methods, you will have just been on a diet, and not a change of lifestyle. This is where most people tend to slip back into their old habits and lose all the hard work they have done. This not only means they have to start again, but they become irritable because they have had to start again. Sometimes, they are also the people who say, "this diet doesn't work" so maybe they should switch to the Mediterranean diet and be happy and comfortable.

That being said, as the Mediterranean diet is not a quick fix but a long-term solution to a healthier and happier you. There are several benefits of following the Mediterranean diet. The small amounts of red wine you are allowed to consume have been shown to give health benefits, as with the healthy oils that you will consume on a daily basis. If followed correctly, you can improve the quality of your heart as what you are aiming to achieve is not just weight loss but a long term healthiness. Some other diets can mainly shock your system and can lead to problems, either by losing weight too quick, of depriving your body of the nutrients it needs to function properly.

Other ways to achieve your objectives is to set yourself goals, many of which will happen naturally because of the food that is allowed on a regular basis.

Examples

Goal 1 - change from full-fat milk to skimmed milk, dairy is limited in the Mediterranean diet so that goal is half way complete.

Goal 2 – Reduce dark meat and switch to white meat, this goal is also nearly completed, as dark meat is limited to maybe once or twice per week The diet even goes further and recommends eating fish or shellfish more than poultry.

Goal 3 – Whole wheat bread instead of white bread; this goal is complete as white bread is to be avoided and only whole grains are to be used.

Goal 4 – Water, even though tea and coffee are allowed, it is recommended to set yourself a goal and reduce the amount of these and switch to herbal tea and water.

Goal 5 – Instead of drinking natural juices, try to eat a piece of fruit, this is more beneficial and will also stop you feeling hungry.

Reward Yourself

If you have reached goals that you set yourself, reward yourself, but not with food. Maybe going out with a friend or something you have wanted to do but put off for another day.

Get Help

If you are you are unsure of how to start or plan your meals, a visit to your doctor may help and they could refer you to a dietician. They will be able to advise on how you should manage your weekly menu.

Heart Smart

There are many things you can do to lead to a healthier heart, some of which you have already covered by switching to a healthier lifestyle and the Mediterranean diet. Using healthier oils, as this limits a number of trans fats in your diet, and eating more fish which are full of omega 3. This is good for your heart and your brain. Exercising the recommended 30 minutes per day, as this will strengthen your heart allowing it to pump blood easier around your body. If you have belly fat, this is directly linked to high blood pressure, so once your belly fat is reducing, your blood pressure should lower too.

There are a few more things that you can do which will improve your heart and also your overall fitness. As with all diets, quitting smoking is beneficial, as this has numerous adverse effects on your heart. Keep quiet about this one...a good night of consensual sex is beneficial to your heart!

A visit to your doctor is not just a good reason to get advice, but you should also have a check-up for blood pressure, blood sugar, and your cholesterol levels. You should find the correct levels for your gender and age group, and if you are not currently in range, find out what you need to do to obtain those levels. Having a starting point is also beneficial because if you have a checkup after a month or two, you will be able to see if anything has changed.

A healthy dose of dark chocolate every now and again can help your heart, as it contains heart-healthy flavonoids which help with inflammation reduction. Try to reduce stress levels, or maybe take a different route home to avoid traffic. If you visit or work in an office block that has an elevator, try taking the stairs instead, because this can be used as one of your exercise quotients or even additional exercise. Switching from your morning and afternoon coffee to a cup of green or black tea, as these have been linked to reducing angina and heart attacks.

If you feel agitated or angry for any reason, instead of letting it build up, go for a long walk. This can lower your stress and lead to your blood pressure dropping, and it is also recommended to walk for at least thirty minutes daily. This can be achieved by parking on the far side of the parking lot if you drive, or even walking to work if you live close. If you travel by bus, just getting off one or two stops earlier can help.

One of the main ways to look after your heart is to keep a positive outlook on life. A 'sunny' outlook is good for your mood and blood pressure, although life may get you down, the newfound health and happiness following the Mediterranean lifestyle will be good for you now, and for many years to come.

Conclusion

I would like to thank you for buying this book and I really hope the information which it contains can be of a great benefit to you. As I have continually mentioned, the Mediterranean diet is not just about the food, it will lead you into a better lifestyle. One where you will feel much better about yourself and feeling much better inside.

It is not the end of the road, just the beginning, actually. Also, with the recipes that are included, you will find new ways of either adapting these or finding new ones...or maybe creating your own. I have given all of my insight to what some people are calling, "The healthiest diet in the world." I would actually stand and say, "I do not really call it a diet" as it is a normal way of life and a normal way of eating. Even if some may argue against it, I am sure there are many people in the Mediterranean who live this life every day, and have a different point of view. Not only do they have a different point of view, they can prove that it works by still being active at a ripe old age to prove it!

23283724R00047

Printed in Poland
by Amazon Fulfillment
Poland Sp. z o.o., Wrocław